Survival Medicine:
Top 15 Plants and Herbs To Survive The Disaster

Table of content

Introduction

While considering the use of medicinal plants, you have to find out the type of injury you have. Various plants are used for the treatment of multiple scenarios, but you have to select a right plant for your injury. You have to find out either you are bleeding or suffering from inflammation. If there is something oozing or you want something for diarrhea. It is essential to get the advantage of the right plant because a wrong medicinal plant can be an invitation to a new problem. Keep it in mind that you can mix plants together to increase their medicinal properties.

If you are having a bite, you may need a drawing agent to remove any toxic substance and an antihistamine to reduce itching. Make sure to be creative, but stay away from dangerous plants. It can be risky for you to use a poisonous plant. With the help of universal edibility test, you can find out ingestible medicinal plants. For instance, boneset is a peculiar plant and you can identify it with its unique look because its stems look pierce through the middle of the leaves. This plant is really fantastic because it can help you to treat flu and cold. Its taste is awful, but it works really well. You can wrap it around your wound to increase the speed of healing. It can be consumed raw or infuse in a tea.

It is a single example, but there are various plants that are really safe and good for medicinal use. It will be good to learn about potential plants found in the wilderness and you can use them as a medicine. This book offers almost 15 herbs and plants that are safe for you and improve your health. You can use them to save the life of any person. Read this book and learn about these plants and herbal medicines:

Chapter 01: Plants and Herbs that can Save Your Life in the Wilderness

Living out in the wild, you'll run over a wide range of therapeutic plants and restorative herbs that can be utilized for various purposes, the length of you know where to look and how to utilize them. Numerous plants are valuable for sustenance, as well as can be utilized as medication also.

Plants can be utilized to mitigate a wide range of illnesses. Everything from skin rash, joint inflammation, cool, fever, looseness of the bowels, headaches, and everything in the middle of can be treated with some sort of plant that can be discovered becoming actually in a wide range of zones. Societies everywhere throughout the world have been utilizing plants for their therapeutic properties for a considerable length of time, much sooner than drug was packaged and sold in pill structure.

Some of the plants and herbs that can be used to safe life in the wilderness are as follows:

Medicinal use

If there is an occurrence of any disease, a specialist's recommendation is undoubtedly best. However, if there is no doctor available, you may need to depend on Mother Nature's abundance for a stretch before you can look for therapeutic consideration. Following are the medicines which nature provides us:

1.   **Aloe Vera:**

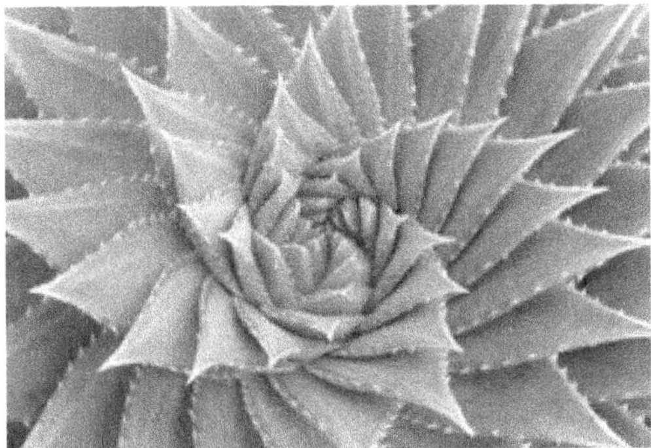

Aloe is a fabulous treatment for skin problems. It is frequently reported that smolders can be mended astoundingly rapidly and the torment diminished rapidly with topical use of Aloe Vera to the blaze zone. And also applying topically, Aloe can likewise be taken inside so it is pretty much as valuable for inner epithelial tissue as it is for the skin. Following are the diseases that Aloe can control:

- Mouth and stomach ulcers

- Lungs and genital tracts.

- Nasal and sinuses

2. Bee Balm:

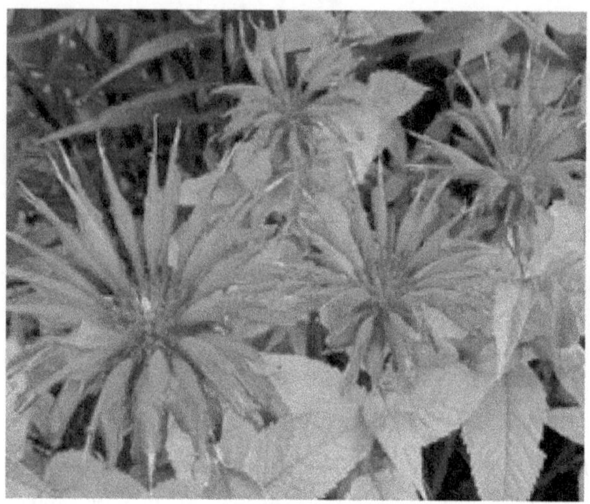

The leaves and flowers of Bee Balm are used for following medicinal purposes:

-       Antiseptic

-       Carminative

-       Diaphoretic

-       Diuretic

Furthermore, it is used to cure following disorders:

-       Colds

-       Headaches

-       Sore throat

- Gastric disorders

- Low fevers

- Insomnia

- Flatulence

- Nausea

- Catarrh

- Menstrual pain

Moreover, steam annihilation of Bee Balm is also very helpful while suffering from cold.

3.   Blackberries

Blackberry leaf is regularly utilized as a therapeutic herb, yet the root has restorative quality. The young shoots are collected in the spring, peeled and utilized as a part of salads. The most astringent part is the root.

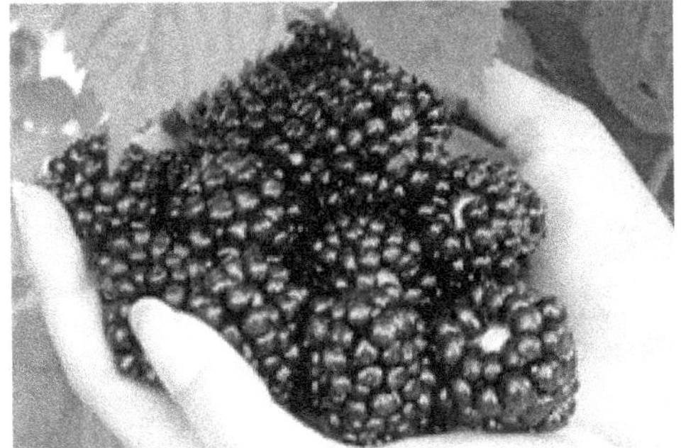

Moreover, they are utilized for the following:

-       Sore throats

-       Mouth ulcers

-       Gum aggravations.

A decoction of the leaves is helpful as a swish in treating thrush furthermore makes a decent broad mouthwash. The nearness of a lot of tannins that give blackberry roots and leaves an astringent impact valuable for treating looseness of the bowels are additionally useful for mitigating sore throats. Moreover, restorative syrup is additionally produced using Blackberry, utilizing the products of the soil bark in nectar for a hack cure.

4.   Boneset

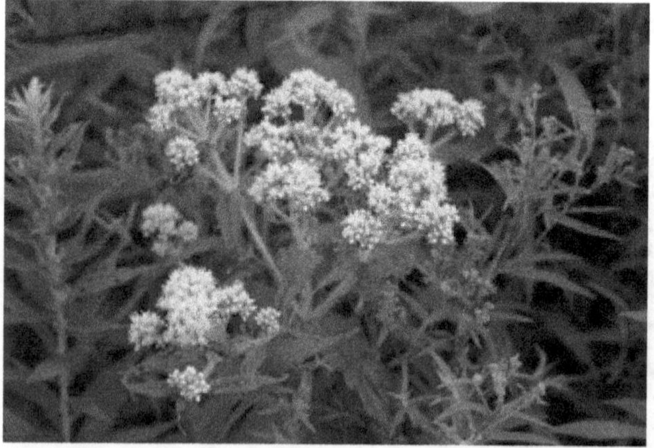

The impact of boneset is slow and persistent. It has great influence on the following:

- Stomach

- Bowels

- Uterus

- Liver

It has been highly regarded as a famous febrifuge, particularly in discontinuous fever, and has been utilized, however less effectively, in typhoid and yellow fevers. It is to a great extent utilized by the Negroes of the Southern United States as a cure in all instances of fever, and in addition for its tonic impacts. As a gentle tonic it is helpful in dyspepsia and general debility, and especially serviceable in the acid reflux of old individuals. The imbuement of 1 OZ of the dried herb to 1 half quart of bubbling water might be taken in wineglassful measurements, hot or icy: for colds and to deliver sweat, it is given hot; as a tonic, frosty.

Food sources:

1.   **Acorns:**

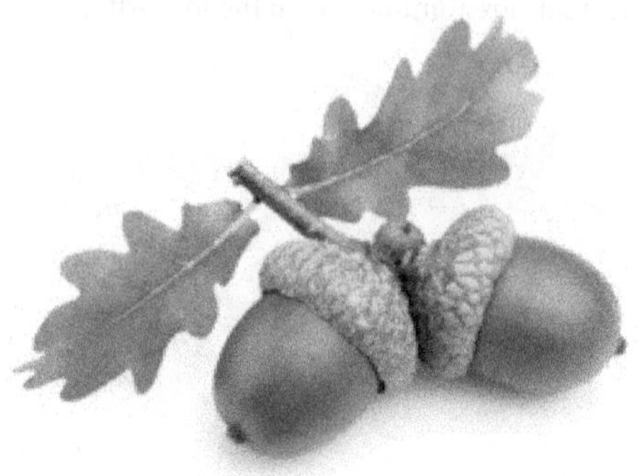

These buds of the oak tree are conventional wellsprings of protein and fat. One can shell and then bubble them, supplanting the water when it becomes brown to dispose of the tannic acid. One might likewise absorb them the running water of a waterway for a day or more

2.   Prickly pear cactus:

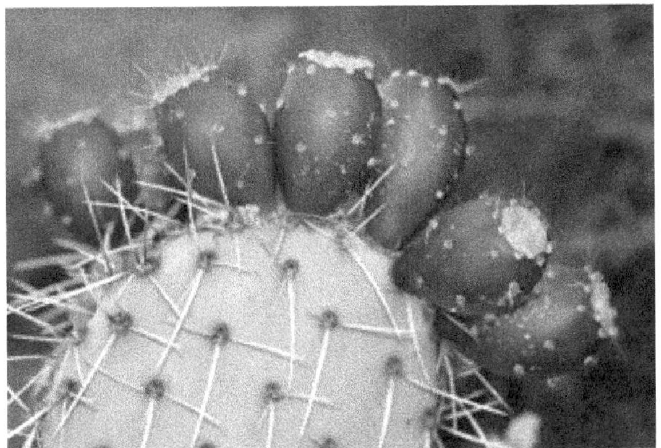

By evacuating the spines and external peel from the youthful stack of the thorny pear, you'll uncover a heavenly and consumable organic product.

3.   Purslane:

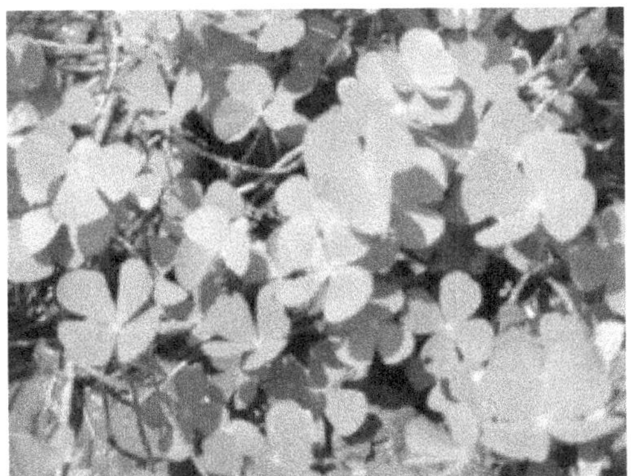

The stems, blossoms, and leaves of this plant contain more omega-3 unsaturated fats than most different greens. Also, here we thought they were just weeds.

Therefore, there are several herbs and plants that can serve the purpose of saving our life in the wilderness. May it as a food resource or as a medicine, plants and herbs can serve the purpose of both.

Chapter 02: Survival Medicine for Fever and Cough

Items produced using botanicals, or plants that are utilized to treat ailments or to keep up the health are called herbal products, botanical items, or phytomedicines. Moreover, the item produced using plants and utilized exclusively for inside use is called a herbal supplement. Furthermore, numerous doctor prescribed medications and over-the-counter prescriptions are additionally produced using plant subsidiaries.

Home grown supplements come in all structures i.e., capsule, dried, powdered, or fluid, and can be utilized as a part of different ways, including:

- Gulped as pills

- Prepared as tea

- Rubbed to the skin as gels

- Added to shower water

The act of utilizing home grown supplements goes back a large number of years. Today, the utilization of home grown supplements is regular among American shoppers. Nonetheless, natural supplements are not for everybody. Since they are not subject to close examination by the FDA, or other representing organizations, the utilization of home grown supplements stays disputable. It is best to counsel your specialist about any indications or conditions you are encountering and to examine the utilization of home grown supplements.

How to cure fever

Many researchers have discovered homemade medicines using herbs and plants that can prove to be useful in curing fever. Some of the approaches that can be used to cure fever are as follow:

1.   In order to avoid dehydration use of fluids to a large number is suggested. To flush the sickness away, herbal teas of following herbs are suggested

-    Chamomile

-    Catnip

-    Peppermint

2.   Moreover, another way used involves the use of elderberries. Syrup is made out of these berries. This syrup, consequently, helps in curing the disease

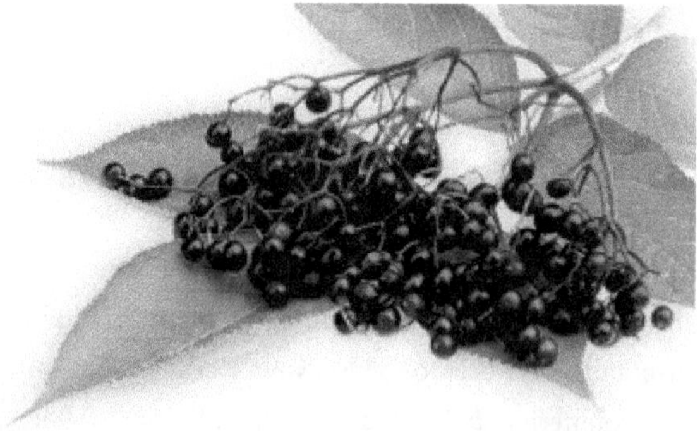

3.   Mix some yarrow tea. Interestingly, this herb opens your pores and triggers the sweating that is said to move a fever toward its end. Steep a tablespoon of herb in some crisply bubbled water for 10 minutes. Let it be cooled. Then, drink a glass or two until you begin to sweat.

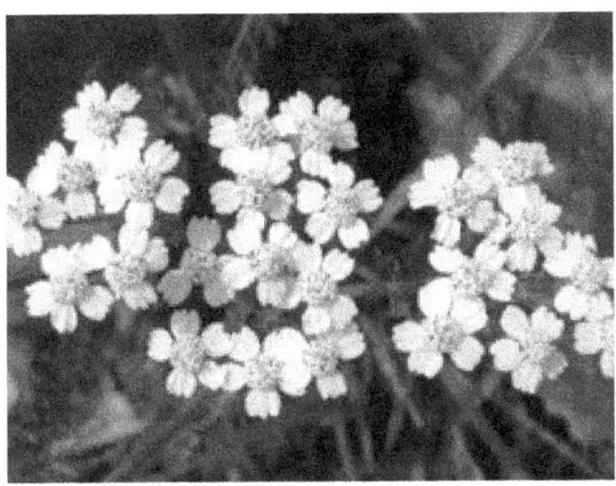

4.   Another herb, elderflower, additionally helps you sweat. Additionally, it happens to be useful for different issues connected with influenza and colds, similar to overproduction of bodily fluid. So, to make elderflower tea, blend two teaspoons of the herb in some bubbled water and let it steep for 15 minutes. Strain out the elderflower. Drink three times each day the length of the fever proceeds.

5.   Drink some hot ginger tea, which likewise actuates sweating. To make the tea, soak a half-teaspoon minced gingerroot in 1 glass simply boiled water. Strain, then drink.

6.   Put some cayenne pepper on your food items whenever you have fever. One of its primary segments is capsaicin, the alarmingly hot fixing that is found in hot peppers. Cayenne makes you sweat furthermore advances fast blood course.

7.   White willow has been utilized for a large number of years by Chinese doctors. A tea made of willow bark is maybe the best-known characteristic treatment for fever and torment. A dynamic compound is salicin, which was confined in 1830 and changed over to aspirin, a standout amongst the most well-known cutting edge drugs. The bitter taste of the willow Bark can be masked with cinnamon, ginger, chamomile, or any of various flavorful herbs

How to cure cold

Before the discovery of anti-biotic, homemade recipes were used in order to cure cold. In order to cure cold following remedial steps must be taken:

1.   Get a lot of liquids. It separates your blockage, makes your throat soggy, and avoids dehydration in your body. The vast majority must drink at least ten to eight ounce glasses of liquid consistently.

2.   You can relax up your stuffy nose while you take in some steam. Hold your head over a jar of boiling water and inhale gradually through your nose. However, care must be taken while you are inhaling steam. Try not to give the warmth a chance to harm your nose. You can likewise get some alleviation with a humidifier in your room. Moreover, attempt to take some relief from a hot shower.

3.   Both saline spray and salt water are used in order to cure cold. In the event that you go the washing course, attempt this formula:

i.   Blend approximately 3 teaspoons of iodide salt and 1 teaspoon of baking soda

ii.   Place the mixture in a sealed shut compartment.

iii.   Now, add 1 teaspoon of the mixture in boiled or refined water.

iv.   Afterwards, fill a syringe with this arrangement and put your head over a bowl. Gently squirt the salt water into your nose. While doing this hold one nostril shut by applying light finger weight while squirting the blend into the other nostril.

v.   Let it deplete for some time and after a few moments treat the other nostril.

vi.   However, be very careful and make use of refined, sterile, or pre-boiled water when you make this arrangement. Or else you may catch a disease.

vii.   Additionally, flush the globule after utilization and leave open to air dry.

Chapter 03: Herbal Antiseptics in the Wilderness

Antiseptic herbs are an operator that slaughters or restrains the development of microorganisms on the outer surfaces of the body and are by and large recognized from natural anti-infection agents that decimate microorganisms inside.

A germicide when connected to wounds and diseases, guarantee that they are perfect and don't deteriorate and have been utilized all through history. A germicide is just a substance that can be put straightforwardly on a slice or contamination to guarantee that it is legitimately spotless and is going to stay perfect as could be expected under the circumstances until the following application.

Germ-killers avoid and balance contamination and the arrangement of discharge by repressing the development of the irresistible life forms. Germs are all around. Some take up habitation in our bodies and benefit us, for example, the amicable microorganisms that colonize the linings of the insides, upper respiratory tract, and lower urinary framework, out-contending terrible organisms, adding to invulnerable safeguard and great processing. Different organisms – infections, microbes, parasites – wreak ruin when they attack our bodies.

Luckily, various herbs have antimicrobial impacts. A considerable lot of these herbs are culinary herbs and flavors, for example, garlic, ginger, thyme, and cinnamon. That implies, regardless of where you will be, you can most likely locate a home grown partner at the neighborhood market. Herbs don't go about as fast or as intensely as medications. For genuine diseases, anti-microbial can spare lives. Then again, herbs produce fewer reactions and don't appear to be connected with the microbial resistance those diseases anti-infection agents.

Various herbs and oils are normal antibacterial and sterile operators and might be utilized as teas, skin washes, made into ointments. Clean herbs will be herbs that contain crucial oils are antibacterial and germ-free. For instance, Thyme is an Antiseptic herb that has been thought about and utilized since old times and the Thymol contained in the herb makes it an astounding germicide and antimicrobial. Numerous individuals are looking to reduce the impacts of artificially based germicides, on their bodies and there are numerous herbs and vital oils that have sterile properties.

Some of the herbal antiseptics that are useful and can help you in the wilderness are as follows:

Cranberry

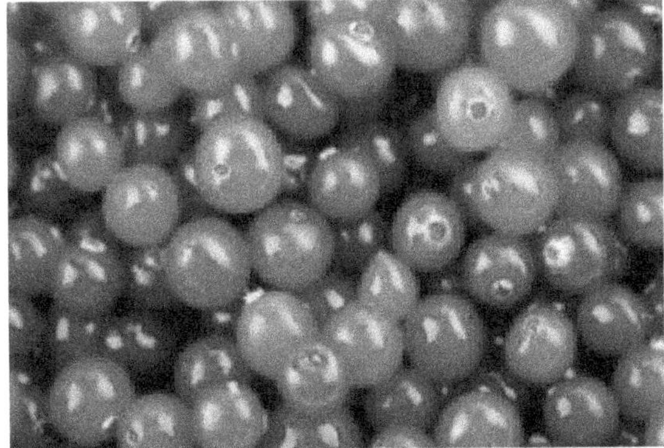

Cranberry also known as Vaccinium macrocarpon is taken as a juice or gathered in tablet structure. It meddles with bacterial adherence to bladder lining, accordingly averting disease. A large portion of the exploration has been in ladies mostly elderly ladies, youthful sexually-dynamic ladies, and pregnant ladies. They are inclined to rehash bladder contaminations. When disease starts, the microbes have effectively connected to the bladder lining. By then, anti-infection agents can clear the contamination quickly and keep microscopic organisms from climbing to the kidneys. For counteractive action, the juice dose utilized as a part of studies reaches from 4 to 32 ounces a day. On the other hand, concentrated juice concentrate can be taken at a dose of one 300-400 milligram tablet, a few times each day. Reactions can incorporate gastrointestinal bombshell. Likewise, concoction constituents of cranberry may hinder the proteins that separate medications, in these way raising blood levels of prescriptions, for instance

-       Coumadin

-       Valium

-       Elavil

-       Motrin, and others

Garlic

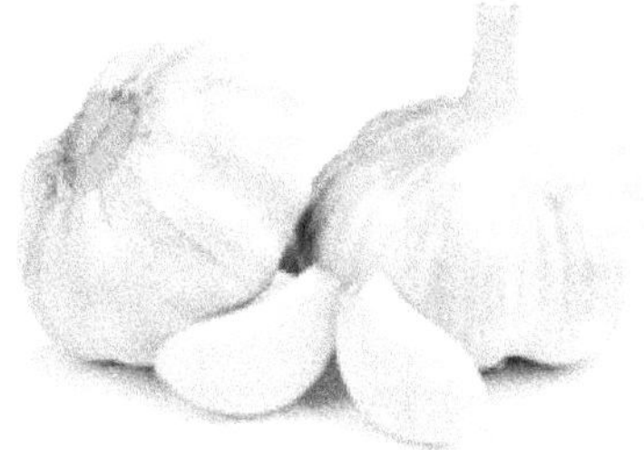

Garlic has antibacterial action against Staphylococcus, Streptococcus, Proteus, Pseudomonas, Mycobacterium, and in addition species connected with loose bowels. However, to some degree strangely, garlic meddles with sickness bringing about microscopic organisms, as opposed to the "amicable" microorganisms, for example, Lactobacillus that colonizes the digestion tracts.

Moreover, garlic is also useful in tackling various species of fungi. Antiviral movement incorporates influenza An and B, rhinovirus, cytomegalovirus, HIV, rotavirus, herpes simplex infection 1 and 2, and a few species that results in pneumonia. According to a particular research those people who use a garlic supplement commencing November through February had few chances of getting sick due to fewer than all those people who use pills. Other Allium types (chives, leeks, onions) have antimicrobial drive as well.

A significant part of the data related to garlic's antimicrobial strength instigates from lab ponders. A smaller amount is thought about in what manner garlic arrangements graft in people contaminated by means of these "bugs." The similar can be assumed in regards to the greater part of alternate herbs recorded beneath. Heat neutralizes garlic's antimicrobial elements. Therefore, it's preeminent to devour it crude or as a pill that promises a specific amount of allicin. On the off chance that you spread over garlic topically as an adhesive, ensure the skin using olive or any other type of oil, spread with dressing or clean material, and evacuate following 60 minutes.

Marshmallow root:

Marshmallow is most normally used to straightforwardness sore throats and dry hacks. The Marshmallow plant contains polysaccharides that have antitussive, adhesive, and antibacterial properties. In light of this, marshmallow soothingly affects aggravated films in the mouth and throat when ingested orally, particularly a sore throat. The antitussive properties diminish dry hacking and avoid further aggravation.

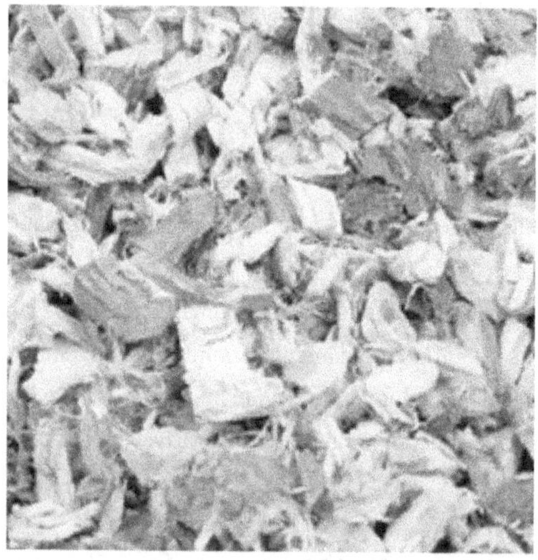

According to the research, marshmallow has been utilized to treat certain digestive issue, including acid reflux, heartburn, ulcerative colitis, stomach ulcers and Crohn's sickness. The system by which it calms sore throats applies to gastrointestinal mucosa too and consistent utilization of marshmallow can help with the agony of ulcerative colitis and Crohn's, and keep stomach ulcers from puncturing. Marshmallow concentrate is now and again added to creams and used to treat provocative skin conditions, for example, dermatitis and contact dermatitis. Extra uses are right now being explored. Marshmallow might be a useful guide to radiologic esophageal examination. There is conditional proof that marshmallow may likewise help with respiratory issue, for example, asthma. Scientists may soon test marshmallow as a characteristic contrasting option to glucose administration in diabetes.

Chapter 04: Common Ailments and Their Herbal Cures

As our way of life is getting techno-astute, we are moving far from nature. While we can't escape from nature since we are a piece of nature. What nature has put away in for us we have not yet completely discovered? This can irritate point with people. Certain European and Oriental nations have been investigating the utilization of herbs and has been by and by since the hundreds of years. Awesome work has been done which escaped the regular man's scope and information .With life on tech-course for each person in the 21st century human sufferings are turning out with various names .The essential herbs have the answer, the general key is no symptoms and powerful cures. The cures are in a state of harmony with nature which is the greatest in addition to point where no other drug can guarantee these actualities. The brilliant certainty is utilization of home grown medicines is autonomous of any age bunches.

Following are some of the common ailments along with their herbal cure are as follows:

Skin problems

1. **Burns:**

i. **Honey:** This is particularly useful for serious smolders. It will stop disease, invigorate skin recovery and keep the blazed region sodden. Nectar is preferred for smolders over about every single medicinal intercession, notwithstanding for severe singeing.

ii. **Prickly pear cactus pads:** Wear gloves to hold the cushions while utilizing a sharp blade to delicately filet the outside skin off the cushions. You will be left with disgusting, oval stack of plant matter. Place the cushions specifically on the smolder and wrap the injury. For sunburn, rub the cushions on the influenced region.

2.   Cuts and scratches.

Each one of us experiences sharp edges may it is a paper cut or a knife cut, regularly again and again. Here's the way to handle the consequences.

i.   **Wound powder:** My natively constructed wound powder stops the dying, dries out the injury, represses disease and empowers recuperating. I by and large utilize a gauze the primary day and afterward leave the injury open a while later

ii.   **Honey:** Stop utilizing the injury powder following a couple days and switch to nectar. It's viable against all known medication safe microscopic organisms and truly speeds recuperating. Simply cover the injury with nectar, swathe, and change the dressing every day.

iii.   **Wound balm:** Use a mix of berberine plants, Siberian elm bark, rosemary leaves, dark walnut bodies, comfrey root, oregano leaves, and dried thyme. Include a quarter-container each of the generally ground herbs to a preparing dish and blend. Spread the mix with around a quarter-inch olive oil, cover the dish, and prepare overnight in a stove on its most reduced warmth setting. In the morning, let the blend cool. Press out and afterward warm the oil. Blend in finely cleaved or ground beeswax — 2 ounces for each measure of mixed oil — and let melt. To check hardness, put a drop of treatment on a plate and hold up until the ointment cools. It ought to stay strong however dissolve following a second of preceding it with your finger.

3.   Rashes:

Rashes come in numerous structures, so medications will shift. Here are a couple of them.

i.   **For hives:** Put on a tincture of Echinacea angustifolia root topically, utilizing a cotton ball to regulate it to the influenced territories. Take a half-teaspoon of the tincture inside every hour or so also.

ii.   **For toxic substance ivy:** Jewelweed balm is ideal. Great added substances are calendula blooms, chamomile blossoms and Siberian elm bark, all of which will calm skin. Include some other herbs you need, however utilize the ethereal parts of a jewelweed plant for half of the dried herbs by weight. At that point, take after the same procedure as above for making the injury treatment.

4.   **Stings and chomps:**

Utilize thorny pear as you would for blazes or Echinacea as you would for hives.

Intestinal Upsets

1.   **Loose bowels:**

Any firmly astringent plant will work for customary looseness of the bowels. Blackberry root, the primary standby utilized for millennia, is greatly compelling. Krameria root, more seasoned pine needles just pulled off the tree, and wild (Geranium maculatum) are all extremely supportive for direction. To utilize, generally slash or crush your preferred dried herb. Add 1 ounce to a quart jug that can take warmth, and load with boiling point water. Spread the invention and let it soak overnight (or for two hours in the event that you truly can hardly wait). Drink it all through the following day. Rehash as required.

2. **Gastric disorder:**

To begin, make juice of 1 beet, 1 bit of green cabbage (about the extent of a medium carrot), 3 carrots, 4 stalks of celery and 4 leaves of crisp plantain (Plantago spp.). Plantain is a typical plant you can generally discover developing in front yards, and is random to the banana of the same name. Cabbage and plantain are the most essential fixings; however they don't taste great without anyone else. Alternate fixings will enhance the taste while helping your adrenal organs, liver and insusceptible framework. Drink this squeeze each morning for breakfast, have cereal for lunch, and have whatever you need for supper. Touchy gut disorder will clear decently quickly on this regimen.

Chapter 05: Precautions to Use Peppers Survival Medicine

To begin with, herbal medicines are used by multiple people which the following purposes:

- Anti-microbial

- Anti-bacterial

- Iodine wash

- Anti-viral

Every measurement of anti-biotic should be weighed deliberately, since re-supply won't come, in the lack of supplies decent homemade information may spare the life of somebody you adore.

Nonetheless, it is important that given the sheer number of home grown meds, and impressive heterogeneity inside and between brands, it is not possible to assess all items for their pharmacology. Albeit some natural pharmaceuticals have had broad examination, a large portion of them have not. Indeed, even those that have been moderately very much concentrated frequently have little data in extraordinary populaces, for example, pediatric, pregnant or lactating ladies, or geriatric populaces, and subsequently, alert ought to be utilized while prescribing natural medications to these populaces.

Some of the side effects of using peppers survival medicine are as follows:

1. **Skin allergies:**

Topical home grown antifungal and antibacterial operators, for example, tea tree oil and lavender are capable of causing rashes or skin disturbance, particularly if utilized at full quality. Before utilizing any topical home grown item, attempt a skin patch test. Place a little measure of the item within the elbow on one arm as it were. Hold up a couple days. On the off chance that the range stays clear, continue with utilizing the home grown item

2. **Dizziness:**

Everybody's body is distinctive, and some individuals are more delicate to herbs than other individuals. Herbs used to treat uneasiness, melancholy and a sleeping disorder may bring about extreme daytime lethargy in specific people. These herbs incorporate chamomile, valerian and kava, with valerian and kava being the in all probability offenders. Abstain from driving or utilizing apparatus until you're certain of the impacts of the herb.

3. **Photosensitivity:**

People taking herbal medicines treat despondency or uneasiness may discover their skin turning out to be more delicate to the sun. They may blaze all the more effortlessly. Commonly, reasonable haired and light-cleaned Caucasians have the most astounding occurrence of photosensitivity, yet this home grown reaction is thankfully uncommon. Common instances of photosensitivity happen when individuals take high dosages of herbal medicine, or take it over a drawn out stretch of time. In the case of taking herbal medicine, maintain a strategic distance from an excess of sun presentation

However, if someone desires to eliminate the danger of getting harmed by using dangerous herbs or plants as medicines, then he must adopt following precautionary measures:

Learn to differentiate between harmful and harmless plants:

Firstly, one must learn how to differentiate between those plants which are harmful and which one of them are harmless. This very approach will help the person choosing the plants for medicinal purposes. If a person is unaware about the plants, then he might get confused and use a wrong herb. This can cause various allergies and can even lead to death

1.   Never utilize any plant without the validness of its character:

Secondly, any plant must not be utilized before its complete recognizable proof. This may represent a risk to one's wellbeing. Hence, a plant must not be utilized before its 100% distinguishing proof

2.   Do not get confused between plants:

Thirdly, multiple plants look similar to one another. However, not all of them are useable. Therefore, never get confused by the deceiving looks of the plant

3.   Avoid excessive use of the herbs:

Fourthly, one should avoid the excessive use of plants and herbs. If one uses the herb in an excessive quantity, then it might cause damage to the person using the herb. In the event that you utilize home grown supplements, take after mark guidelines deliberately and utilize the endorsed dose as it were. Never surpass the suggested dose, and search out data about who ought not to take the supplement.

4.   Look for reactions:

If any symptoms, for example, sickness, unsteadiness, cerebral pain, or furious stomach, happen, diminish the measurements or quit taking the home grown supplement

5.   Be ready for an unfavorably responses:

A serious hypersensitive response can bring about trouble relaxing. If any unlikely event occurs, rush to the emergency to avoid any harm.

6.   Do some research:

Research about the organization whose herbs you are taking. All home grown supplements are not made equivalent, and it is best to pick a respectable maker. Moreover, following things must be checked before using any homemade medicine:

-       Has the manufacturer put some effort in developing the herbal product or if he is employing the some one's research.

-       Does the item make abnormal or difficult to demonstrate claims?

-       Does the item mark give data about the institutionalized equation, reactions, fixings, bearings, and safeguards?

-       Is the provided data clear and simple to peruse?

Conclusion

To put in a nutshell, plants and herbs are an efficient source of medicines. This book will expound upon all of those perspectives that will help an individual and guide him about the herbal medicines. Moreover, living out in the wild, you'll keep running over an extensive variety of remedial plants and helpful herbs that can be used for different purposes, the length of you know where to look and how to use them. Various plants are profitable for sustenance, and can be used as pharmaceutical too. Plants can be used to alleviate an extensive variety of ailments. Everything from skin rash, joint irritation, cool, fever, detachment of the insides, cerebral pains, and everything amidst can be treated with some kind of plant that can be found turning out to be really in an extensive variety of zones. Social orders all over the place all through the world have been using plants for their helpful properties for an impressive time span, much sooner than medication was bundled and sold in pill structure. Regardless, it is essential that given the sheer number of home developed meds, and great heterogeneity inside and between brands, it is unrealistic to evaluate all things for their pharmacology. But some normal pharmaceuticals have had wide examination, an extensive part of them have not. Surely, even those that have been decently especially focused as often as possible have little information in remarkable peoples. Therefore, the book includes in itself all the precautions that are necessary

FREE Bonus Reminder

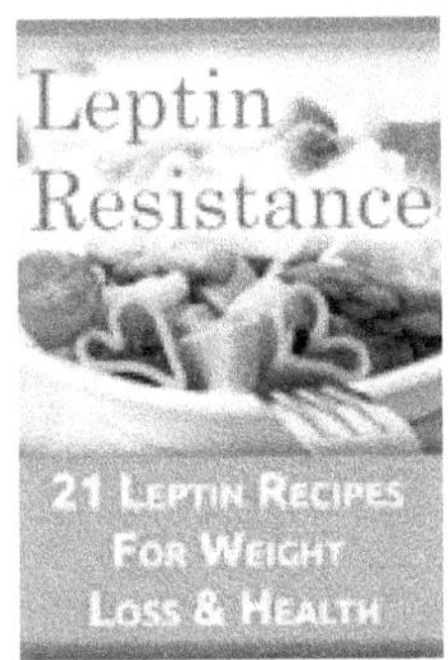

If you have not grabbed it yet, please go ahead and download your special bonus report *"Leptin Resistance. 21 Leptin Recipes For Weight Loss & Healthy Living"*.

Simply Click the Button Below

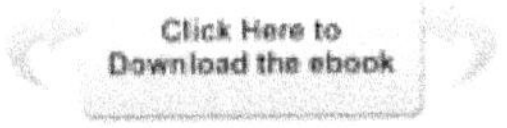

OR **Go to This Page**

http://easyweightlossway.com/free/

BONUS #2: More Free & Discounted Books

Do you want to receive more Free & Discounted Books?

We have a mailing list where we send out our new Books when they go free or with a discount on Kindle. Click on the link below to sign up for Free & Discount Book Promotions.

=> **Sign Up for Free & Discount Book Promotions** <=

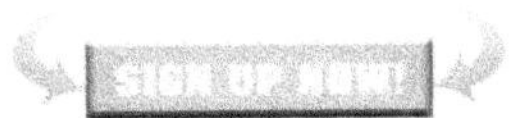

OR Go to this URL

http://zbit.ly/1WBb1Ek

www.ingramcontent.com/pod-product-compliance
Lightning Source LLC
Chambersburg PA
CBHW050804240726

48654CB00008B/630